This book contains two book manuscripts authored by Sammy Parker:

Book 1: Depression: Naturally Free Yourself of Depression and Heal Anxiety, Panic Attacks, and Stress

Book 2: How to Analyze People Using Human Psychology to Successfully Analyze and Understand Anyone from Anyplace and Anywhere

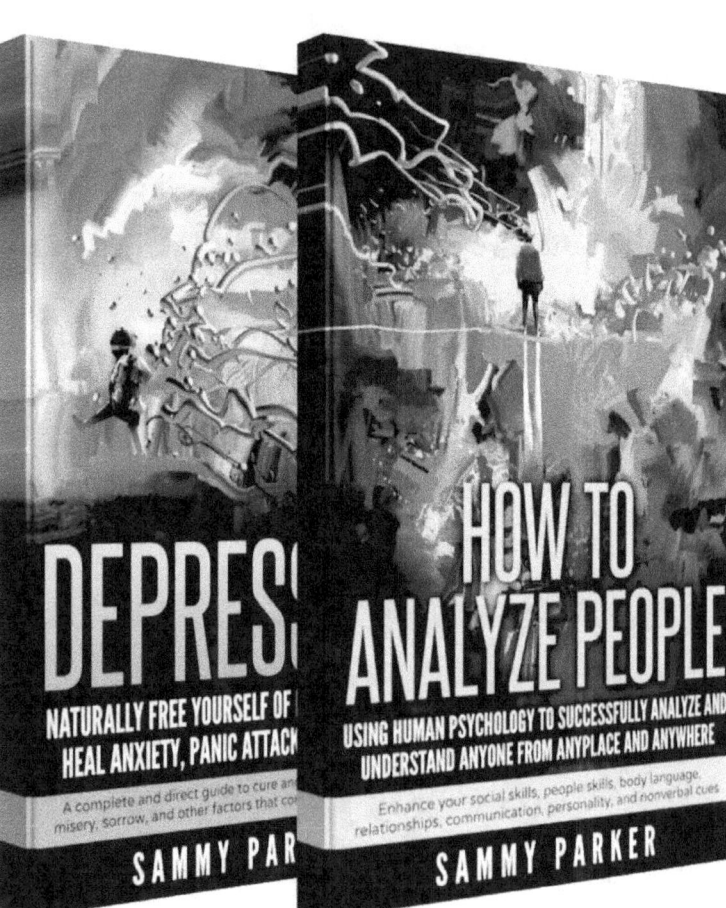

DEPRESS

NATURALLY FREE YOURSELF OF
HEAL ANXIETY, PANIC ATTACK

A complete and direct guide to cure an
misery, sorrow, and other factors that con

SAMMY PAR

HOW TO
ANALYZE PEOPLE

USING HUMAN PSYCHOLOGY TO SUCCESSFULLY ANALYZE AND
UNDERSTAND ANYONE FROM ANYPLACE AND ANYWHERE

Enhance your social skills, people skills, body language,
relationships, communication, personality, and nonverbal cues

SAMMY PARKER

Depression: Naturally Free Yourself of Depression and Heal Anxiety, Panic Attacks, and Stress

A Complete and Direct Guide to Cure and Overcome Sadness, Misery, Sorrow and Other Factors that Contribute to Depression

BY SAMMY PARKER

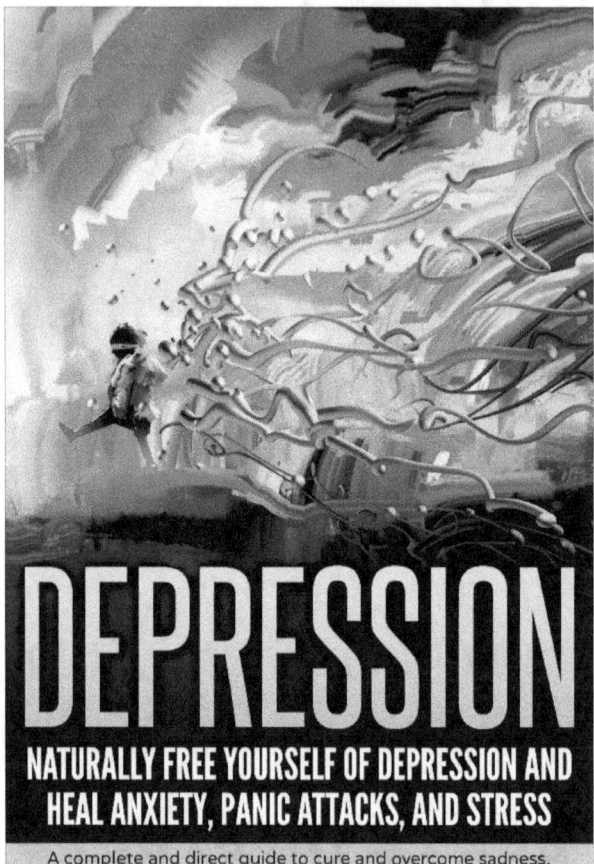

DEPRESSION

NATURALLY FREE YOURSELF OF DEPRESSION AND HEAL ANXIETY, PANIC ATTACKS, AND STRESS

A complete and direct guide to cure and overcome sadness,
misery, sorrow, and other factors that contribute to depression

SAMMY PARKER

Preview of this book

Depression can encompass feelings that can include sorrow, misery, sadness, anger, lethargy, and many more. These feelings are related to a disorder, sometimes even a disease or illness within your body.

You are also going to gain insight into the myths of depression. There are common misconceptions that hinder your treatment, as well as do's and don'ts that might be stopping you from gaining proper treatment.

Uncover:

1. How depression affects your life

2. How to boost your self-esteem

3. A care plan to start taking action

4. New discovered, researched, and proven techniques

You are going to discover who the best person to help you will be, so that you can find fulfillment in your life. You might be surprised at who can truly help you the most. Take the journey now. Start your recovery and battle with depression today.

Table of Contents for Depression: Naturally Free Yourself of Depression and Heal Anxiety, Panic Attacks, and Stress

Introduction

Depression affects an estimated 350 people worldwide. People of all ages suffer from depression, including children and retired adults. Depression is also considered the leading cause behind disability on a global scale. Statistics from the World Health Organization show that fewer men suffer depression versus men. Depression can lead to suicide, unless someone seeks the help they need or helps their loved one get the help they need.

Depression is a chronic condition, with long-lasting or severely intense negative emotions. Depression can lead to additional health conditions. It is also a condition that can greatly affect your work, school, and relationships.

More than 800,000 people die each year as a result of suicide, driven by depressive emotions. Suicide due to depression is the second highest cause of death in 15 to 29 year olds, according to the World Health Organization (2016).

If you are one of the 350 million people who suffer from depression, you now know that you are not alone. You have a medical and psychological condition that can be managed with various treatment plans.

You have to be willing to get the help you need or help your loved one see that they can get the treatment they need. There are barriers to proper treatment. It resides in the improper health care system throughout the world, even in developed countries.

A World Health Assembly met in 2013 to focus on the rise of depression among people in the world. This assembly has opened up new pathways for you to gain the treatment and help you need. Many states are now offering free visits to psychologists for low income families. Health insurance has started to add treatment for depression, at least on a minimal basis.

Whether you are a teenager or a senior citizen, you also have tools at your disposal to gain the help you require. This complete and direct guide will help you cure your depression, overcome your anxiety and stress, and get rid of the sadness you feel.

You will be able to have healthy relationships, built on self-confidence, as well as regain your health. Discover what you can do to heal yourself, as well as gain help from others to help you heal. You never know what resources are going to be available to you, until you try.

You are a strong person. You are capable of healing your mind. Take action now and discover how you can eliminate your depression.

I want you to take special attention to chapter 8. This chapter is important because it provides up to date research and techniques that can be used to treat your depression. The main goal of this book is to not only help you understand why you have depression, but also give you a new and holistic views and ideas that are currently present within the past 3 years. I hope this book provides a ton of value to your life and to the lives of others. Thank you!

Chapter 1: Historical View of Depression

Depression is not a new disorder. Historical documents provide us with a pattern of evidence suggesting that depression has always been a health issue for humans. Healers, writers, and philosophers have written about depression, the struggles people have gone through, and ways to treat the illness.

In these historical documents, depression was referred to as melancholia. The first known, written, reference to this disorder was from a 2nd millennium BC Mesopotamian text. During the early centuries, and to a certain degree now, depression and other mental disorders were thought to be demonic possession, thus priests would attend to the "victims" of the disorder.

Physical injuries were handled by physicians, but depression was not considered a physical illness. It was thought of as a spiritual illness. Greek and Roman doctors in later centuries began to think of depression as a biological and psychological disorder. These doctors started prescribing massage, gymnastics, music, special diets, and baths as a cure. They also included a concoction with donkey's milk and poppy extract.

Hippocrates was one of the most famous physicians who attribute depression to personality traits and mental illness as an imbalance of the body fluids. At the time he believed it was an imbalance of black bile, yellow bile, blood, and phlegm. Hippocrates listed mania, phrenitis, and melancholia as mental illnesses. Phrenitis was a brain fever. Hippocrates was the doctor who prescribed bloodletting as a way to treat the imbalance of fluids and to heal depression.

Cicero, a Roman philosopher, had a different opinion. Cicero believed melancholia was due to rage, grief, and fear. His opinion was that depression was not physical, but mental.

More Modern Explanations

In more recent centuries, Robert Burton (1621), wrote the Anatomy of Melancholy. He ascribed depression to psychological and social causes. He felt that fear, poverty, and solitude led to depression. His solution was exercise, diet, travel, distraction, cleansers, herbal remedies, bloodletting, music, and marriage.

The 18th and 19th centuries were a larger change in the thoughts of mental illnesses and depression. The "Age of Enlightenment" listed depression as an unchangeable weakness, one that was inherited, and affected people were shunned. In many cases, they were locked away in institutions and forgotten, (Mental Help, 2007).

Psychology and the understanding of depression have come a long way since the early centuries, even since the early 1900s. Even through the 1950s, mental disorders, including depression were not talked about. If someone suffered from a disorder they were either put in an institution or left at home locked away from visitors.

Psychology started taking a more active, research role, in the 60s and 70s. Aaron Beck developed a new theory about depression in the 60s. He stated depression was caused by negative thinking patterns, where one would think about themselves, their future, and the world.

Other research was working on depression as an endogenous or neurotic reaction. As an endogenous condition, a person would suffer from a biological condition that caused the signs and symptoms of depression. A neurotic or reactive reaction was caused by stressful events.

It was discovered in the 1950s that a chemical imbalance affected the body and brain, leading to depression. Two chemicals in the body caused the imbalance: reserpine and isoniazid. These two chemicals would alter neurotransmitter levels, bringing depressive symptoms to the forefront.

Further work was conducted, where a separation of bipolar disorder and depression were made. In the mid-1970s, a new term was coined—Major Depressive Disorder (Wikipedia, 2016).

Major Depressive Disorder, along with melancholia are listed in the DSM VI versions. Psychology and doctors are still trying to gain a full understanding of depression; however, most understand it is either a chemical imbalance or psychological disorder brought about my fear and anxiety.

Chapter 2: Discover the Cause of Your Depression

Treatment of depression is only possible, when you have an understanding of the cause of your depression. There are main causes of depression that can bring about a temporary condition or one that lasts for one's lifetime. If you are tired of battling your depression, then seek the advice of a physician and psychologist to determine the root cause.

The following are key factors that may lead to depression:

- Abuse

- Medications

- Personal conflicts

- Death or loss

- Genetics

- Major events

- Social isolation

- Illness

- Substance abuse

- Medical disorders

Abuse

Abuse can be sexual, violence, or mental. When inflicted upon a person that person may begin to feel depressed. They start to lose their self-confidence and self-esteem.

Medications

Specific medications prescribed for health issues, such as high blood pressure, can contain beta-blockers. Reserpine can also be included in certain medications.

Both beta-blockers and reserpine can increase the risk of depression in the person taking the medication.

Personal Conflicts

Personal conflicts among friends, family, and co-workers can lead a person to feel depressed, unable to handle the disputes, and unable to face their life.

Death or Loss

The loss of a loved one naturally creates feelings of depression. These feelings can be short lived or may require additional help. It is a mental situation for the person because of their emotions.

Genetics

Studies have found that a family history of depression may link to reserpine and other chemical imbalances, thus a cause can be one's genetic makeup. Depression does not have to link with a genetic disorder for a steady family history of the illness. It can also be linked to the imprinting on the child. A young child may grow up with depression because their main character suffers from it. The exact cause of a family history of depression is still unknown, but there are physical and psychological causes researchers have studied.

Major Events

Major events in your life can be a direct cause of your depression. Marriage, moving, losing a job, getting divorced, losing income, retiring, graduating, obtaining a new job, or suffering from combat can lead to depression.

Social Isolation

Social isolation due to another mental illness, physical illness, or other reason can be a cause of depression. If a person feels like an outcast, there is a potential that the person can feel depressed. Moving away from this isolation or the disparaging remarks can often help a person recover.

Substance Abuse

Substance abuse can be a cause of depression or it can be the result of depression. Approximately 30% of people who suffer from substance abuse issues have also been diagnosed with depression, (Medicine Net, n.d.).

Medical Disorders

Illness, such as cancer, can lead to depression. The reaction to the illness, the feeling that life is over, and the medications required to treat the illness have often been the cause of depression in patients.

The following medical disorders are known to cause depression in patients. These disorders are not as likely to be seen as the cause of depression, and yet for millions of people they can be.

Alzheimer's and Dementia

Patients who are diagnosed with a type of dementia are often suffering from depression. Their confidence begins to dwindle as their memory becomes faulty. They also feel unsettled and worried. Fear and anxiety can lead to depressive symptoms. For some, depression may be the first sign of a brain disorder, such as dementia. Dementia and its various forms, is caused by a shrinking of the brain, which affects mood, memory, and overall cognition.

Thyroid

Thyroid, including Grave's Disease, hyper, and hypo thyroid conditions are an imbalance with a person's hormones. The hormones: TSH, T3, and T4 can become over or under produced. When this occurs, the brain function is affected. There can be short-term memory loss and pseudo-dementia symptoms. When the hormones are corrected, the brain returns to normal function, and depression can be eliminated.

Menopause and PMS

Both are hormonal conditions that have been linked to temporary depression. When the hormone production changes a person can start to feel bad about themselves, feel fatigued, and show other signs of depression. A correction of the hormone production alleviates the troubles.

Chapter 3: Signs and Symptoms

Approximately 10 symptoms are common in people with depression. These common symptoms are not all inclusive. You do not need to have all of them to be considered "clinically" depressed. A diagnosis should be made by a mental health professional or your physician.

Symptoms

- Fatigue

- Concentration difficulty

- Guilt

- Worthless or helpless feelings

- Insomnia, excessive sleeping or early-morning wakefulness

- Restlessness

- Irritability

- Loss of interest

- Appetite changes

- Persistent aches and pains, digestive issues

- Anxiousness, sadness, or an empty feeling

- Thoughts of suicide, or an attempt

These symptoms can occur with physical disorders. For example, a person with a thyroid disorder can feel many of these symptoms, but have a root cause based in a hormonal imbalance. Correcting the hormonal imbalance can adjust a person's way of thoughts and "cure" these depressive symptoms.

Issues can also arise from other mental disorders. Anxiousness, irritability, restlessness, and appetite changes have been caused by social anxiety or other fears.

When the majority of these symptoms are present, then depression is usually the diagnosis, but remember to check for underlying causes.

Warning Signs of Depression

A person who is suddenly very calm or happy after being extremely sad, may have depression.

An individual who always thinks about death or is talking about death may suffer from depression.

With clinical depression, the symptoms become worse, with more trouble sleeping, eating, sadness, or a loss of interest and concentration.

Some people with depression take more risks. These risks are usually based on death, such as driving without headlights, hiking without proper equipment, or being in other situations that could lead to an "accidental" death.

Depression can make you lose interest in relationships and those you truly care about.

You may often be making statements about feeling helpless, hopeless, or worthless. Your self-confidence is at an all-time low. You may feel like people are disrespecting you, treating you incorrectly, or that it is your entire fault because you are worth nothing.

Many people show signs of depression and suicidal thoughts, when they get their life in order. They might change their will or tie up loose ends in preparation of dying.

Talk about dying or killing one's self is not always seen, but in the last days before an attempt is made more of this talk happens. Unscheduled visits or calling people that a person loves can be a sign of suicidal thoughts.

Statements, such as "I want out," or "It is better if I was not here," are usually signs of depression, where the person is getting closer to suicide (Webmd, n.d.).

Hiding Symptoms

Depression takes over slowly. Sometimes a person does not realize they suffer from depression, until their loved one points out the numerous changes in their behavior, relating to the above symptoms.

Other individuals are aware that there are problems, but they ignore the issues or think they can deal with it on their own. This type of person is bound to hide their feelings and symptoms until there is truly no possible way to hide them.

It can be easier if the clinical depression is in a mild form or is a result of a known cause like a recent death in the family. It is also possible that the person has hidden their symptoms for many years due to a high level of self-control, yet they have dangerous thoughts.

Observation is one of the best ways for you to determine if a person around you is hiding their depression symptoms.

If you feel you might have depression, there are things you can do. You can start to track your behavior in a journal. If you already write in a journal, back track and see if you have sudden mood shifts or dark thoughts.

Chapter 4: Depression Misconceptions

Depression like many mental illnesses is seen in the wrong light. These misconceptions can hinder you from getting the help you need. It can also make it difficult for you to understand the disease.

Myths

- **Depression and sadness are the same**. Sadness is a symptom of depression; however, you can be sad without being affected by depression. Sadness can result from a deep, powerful memory. When you think of this memory, you can feel sad, but it is not a constant feeling. Depression is a chronic condition, where sadness is just one of the negative emotions swirling in your brain. The feeling also sucks the life out of you, making daily life arduous.

- **Depression is a sign of mental instability/weakness**. There is a stigma attached to all mental illnesses, including depression. Most people decide to remain quiet about their suffering because of the stigma. The truth is, no one asks to feel depressed, sad, and upset. Depression affects people of all social, psychological, and biological types—not just a specific type of person.

- **It occurs because of a traumatic event**. Yes, there are certain events, which can trigger depression. However, not everyone suffering from depression has gone through a traumatic event. Loving a loved one, being in combat, or going through a divorce can lead to depression. There are feelings of remorse, sadness, emptiness, and loneliness for a period of time. These symptoms may last, without help, for months, even years. Yet, they can also be alleviated within a few weeks.

- **It's all in your mind**. Emotional symptoms do result based on feelings; however, insomnia, fatigue, appetite change, chest pains, and chronic muscle aches can also be an issue. Depression is not just a mental situation, but a physical one, when it goes on long enough.

- **Depression is not a real illness**. Depression is not going to fit one treatment plan, but it does not mean it is not a medical condition that does not require treatment. The Mayo Clinic states that hormone imbalances, the brain, and neurotransmitters that are affected by depression make depression a true illness. It affects a person on various levels.

- **Men don't suffer depression**. The thought that a "real" man will not suffer from depression, is yet another myth. Anyone can be affected by depression. Yes, studies show more women than men suffer from depression, but men still have a higher rate of suicide due to depressive symptoms than women. A middle-aged white male is more at risk for suicide, according to studies. A reason for this myth, is that men tend to have a different way of expressing the problem and thus depression in men is more easily overlooked.

- **All depression is genetic**. Only 10 to 15 percent of people in the world, with a history of family depression will have depression. While it may be hereditary or at least a learned behavior through childhood, it does not mean that if one or both parents are depressive that you will suffer from the same. You do need to be aware and have your levels checked for a chemical imbalance, but this is for peace of mind versus a high risk of developing depression.

- **Medication is the only cure and you need it all your life**. Medication is not the only way to treat your depression. If you do need medication for your depression, you may not need it your entire life. Medication is a short-term requirement. About 40 percent of people with depression use psychotherapy with great results versus medication. Yes, medication can help improve your moods for a time, but your body can also become used to the same medicine, lowering its effects.

- **Discussing your depression makes it worse**. Kids tend to feel this is true, more than adults. Kids feel if they talk about their depression, their feelings will only become worse because those around them will not understand. Adults can also feel this way or feel that talking does not help because they are forced to admit to all the problems they have. In fact, talking about one's feelings is a way to proactively work on positive reinforcement, versus the negative, destructive feelings that rule when you hide your emotions (Hall, 2014).

Knowing these are myths and what the truths are, you can start to focus on your treatment and combat depression in the best possible way for you. There are some Do's and Don'ts that can help you with your depression that also go along with these myths.

Do's

- You do want to recognize that depression can lead to other health issues.

- You want to take steps to minimize other health issues by eating correctly and exercising often.

- It is necessary to develop a way for you to handle stress.

- Get a medical opinion regarding your symptoms and determine if there is an underlying cause of your depression.

- Do understand that medications are only a small help, and there are better treatment options.

Don'ts

- Don't avoid your feelings. Seek treatment.

- Don't settle. You can gain treatment; you don't have to "live" with your moods.

- Don't treat just the depression, look for other causes and determine if there is something else affecting you.

- Don't let inactivity and listlessness win. Make yourself go for a walk.

- Don't neglect the signs you see in yourself. Speak out.

Writing these do's and don'ts is easy. Pushing yourself to follow them and lead a better life is the hard part, but not impossible.

Nothing is impossible, if you try hard enough to face what ails you. Without following through, you could be placing yourself in more danger. Depression can lead to obesity, diabetes, heart attacks, chronic digestive issues, and suicide. Take step after step and work your way to a depression free life. You can do it.

Chapter 5: How Depression Affects Different Aspects of your Life

Depression not only affects you, but it affects various aspects of your life, including the people you love. Discovering how your life is affected by depression can be one more step towards making improvements and pushing you towards the help you need.

Many times we lose sight of those around us, the love we have for them, and how they can help us, when suffering from depression. Reminding yourself that you do have people who care and they are willing to be "bothered" by your troubles will help you in your treatment.

It is true that you will get into a vortex of limited sight when you are in the midst of depression. This cycle of negative thinking can battle between knowing people will help you if you ask, and being unable to ask. Perhaps you have had thoughts that they will not be able to help you or understand. Maybe, you have tried to reach out, but their own lives are busy and you feel like you are just in the way.

There might be times when you've thought, "I'm always the one to get a hold of that person(s), so obviously they do not care about me." Often the other side to the story is that your friends and family do care, but you are right—they are living their life and sometimes that life is just as bad as yours.

Your friends might be battling their own depression. It's even happened to me. I was suffering greatly from depression brought on by the loss of a loved one, although that loved one was not completely gone, his mind was due to dementia. My friend's said they would be there, but never called. It turned out that one of my friends was suffering from post-partum depression and another had been battling depression for 10 years. All three of us didn't tell each other of our struggles and battles with depression, but tried to keep it all inside. Instead of leaning on those that could help and understand, we all chose to keep it to ourselves and try to deal with it in their own way.

The relationships could have been completely and forever fractured. Some relationships were among the friends because of the depression and mistakes made. For example, one friend lost their spouse in a divorce due to the severe depression plaguing the friend.

Relationships and Depression

Each side has a view. This view may be in line with the other side or it might be completely different, and somewhere in the middle is the truth to everything. Depression and relationships are like this.

You are in a dark place. Everything you see around you is negative. The things that should be bringing you happiness are not. You also feel that no one can understand. You tend to withdraw. There is also a high likelihood that you are complaining about many things to yourself and to your friends. Every little thing can be a complaint, when depression has its hooks in you.

The deep relationships you have are often able to deal with this side of you. Their love demands that they help you work through the troubles, at least for a time. Those who love you want the best, they want to be able to fix your problems, but their own problems can start to stack up. They can begin to affect the person, so they are unable to help you.

If it gets to be too much or you are too unwilling to seek help, then the loved one may pull away. They may try to seek happiness elsewhere or simply give up on you. The strength that exists in your relationship will determine whether a person is willing to stay by your side, through the tough times and provide the care you need.

Some relationships are not strong enough. Sometimes divorce or avoidance is the only way your loved one can handle the depressive state you are in. People tend to seek happiness, when surrounded by unhappiness. They don't want to feel as sad and depressed as you. If they struggle with their own depression, then they may also pull away.

Since depression often means sleeping a lot, stopping the hobbies you used to love, and having a lack of concentration, relationships are often the first to be harmed. A person with depression may refuse to do anything that used to be enjoyable, leaving the one in the relationship without depression to wonder why the person is pulling away. It is a cycle that can injure relationships forever.

The one truth is that the person you love does not want to pull away. They do not want to seek a different relationship, but at some point they are going to realize that they are either enabling your depressive state or they are unable to help you because it is hurting them.

A caregiver, even one that loves you and is there for you, has to take care of themselves and their needs before they can help you.

Health

Relationships are not the only area of your life to suffer. Medically, your mind is a powerful tool capable of many things, including making you sick. Depression may be a manifestation of your negative emotions, but it can be expressed in severe, chronic pain.

If there is no underlying health condition causing your depression like thyroid disorder, you can make your back, head, or your entire body ache. You can make yourself feel ill, as if you have some horrible disease, and yet have depression. This pain makes you want to ignore the fun things you use to do in life. You might even wish to lay in bed all day because of the pain and yet, this will not provide a release of the pain.

Depression can also bring on IBS symptoms. Perhaps irritable bowel syndrome is actually more prevalent because of the high rate of depression. This is unknown, but one thing is for certain—when you suffer from depression your insides suffer.

People with depression have reported IBS with diarrhea. Their stomach becomes so upset, it gets nauseous, and requires many bathroom trips. Each time you have this issue, you are hurting your body even more. You can start developing ulcers and hemorrhoids.

Work

Work is greatly affected, whether you show up or not. First, if you do go to work or speak with co-workers when you telecommute, you are often negative. You also tend to avoid doing your job. If you have deadlines, you start missing these deadlines. The quality of your work suffers, and eventually, you are seen as not performing your duties correctly. This can lead to you losing your job.

If you admit to the depression, then you have an out, but only for a short time. Your boss or bosses will only care for a short time that you have a problem. They will still want to see you returning to a proper performance level.

Depression can also be a hindrance for you going to work at all. There are times when a person with depression calls in sick or requests more time off than they are paid for. These constant call-ins usually lead to attendance issues, and companies tend to have a policy of "excessive" call-ins. You can be put on notice that one more missed day in a certain time period will be the end of your job.

Chapter 6: Techniques to Boost Your Self-Esteem

Self-esteem is one area that is greatly affected by depression. It can also be a cause of depression. There are techniques you can use to boost your self-esteem. These techniques do not work for everyone with depression as it does have a lot to do with the level of severity. However, working on these techniques can start to help you in numerous ways. Setbacks are okay; it is when you give up that you are hurting yourself and others.

1. Positive self-talk is the hardest thing for someone with depression. A journal can be a helpful tool. Each morning or every night before bed, write down one positive aspect of your day or about yourself. Even one positive thought can help you change what you are feeling. It may not last more than 10 minutes, but the fact that you are retraining your brain to focus on the positive for a short time, will start to become a routine.

    A routine got you into the negative thinking you do, so a new routine of positive thoughts for a short time can get you out of it. Positive talk about yourself is also a way to feel good about who you are.

2. You should not compare yourself to someone else. It can be hard. You have all these people around you and they seem to have a "perfect" world. The trouble is, you are often misled into thinking their world is perfect. Like you, people hide the true nature of their life. It is possible for someone to be depressed, even more depressed than you and not show it.

Another person might have many money worries and constantly be fighting with their spouse before a divorce happens suddenly. Comparing yourself to another is going to make you feel bad about yourself, and a lot of what you see isn't the reality.

3. Perfection is something you must let go. You cannot reach perfection because the world is not perfect. Is a mountain perfect? Is a tree? No. Even a symmetrical building can have something that is slightly off. As the human race, no one is perfect no matter how much we try. By continuing to try, you are hurting yourself. Let the control fall away and live life.

4. Exercise is known to release happy endorphins. These endorphins help you feel good about yourself because you are doing something to

improve yourself. When self-esteem and depression are combined, it is very difficult for you to choose to exercise.

It takes a lot of drive, even if you pay to use a fitness center. But, every time you exercise you are going to feel energized, better about yourself, and have the endorphins to feel happy. Exercise also helps you keep your health.

5. If you make a mistake move on. Our brains tend to overanalyze mistakes. One trick that has been learned is to choose music that helps you feel peaceful. For example, ocean waves for deep sleep, is a channel on streaming radios. This channel offers various soft piano music and ocean wave sounds. Sometimes there are also birds chirping.

These sounds can help your body and mind relax, giving you the opportunity to tell your brain you are not going to think about the mistakes you made for the day. A lot of building your self-esteem and ending your depression is in telling yourself you are not "going to dwell on the bad," and will think of a positive thought.

6. Self-esteem requires that you start doing things you enjoy. Depression stops you from doing

what you enjoy, and yet the solution to both depression and self-esteem is to get back into your hobbies. If you need to have a friend help you with this. You might be hesitant to go out, but the right friend will push you to.

7. Always give yourself a reward, even for the small accomplishments you have done. For example, if you have written 10,000 words in a book, celebrate it. It might not be the whole book, but at least you reached a milestone.

8. Start focusing on the things you can change about yourself or the situation you are in. If you feel down because of money, go back to school, get a second job, or change careers.

Increasing your self-esteem will take time. Depression can get in the way of progress, but accept that, move on from it, and keep plugging away at changing yourself and soon depression may start to correct itself.

Chapter 7: Treatment for Depression

Treatment for depression comes in many forms. One of these treatment forms may be suitable for you. However, know that researchers are also working on new approaches to treating depression that may be better suited for you.

Drugs

Medications are a temporary cure for depression. Medications are something you can build a intolerance to. They can also cause more depression in you, depending on your body and mind.

Some individuals who have taken anti-depressants actually feel more fatigue and suicidal. Citalopram is a common anti-depressant given for depression. Reports indicate that 30% of people on this medication find they are used to it within a few months and their symptoms are no longer being taken care of. Medications can also lead to addictions and health issues. Most anti-depressants have a long list of side effects, do's and don'ts that are not good for you.

Therapy

Numerous types of therapy exist. Cognitive behavior therapy (CBT) is the most common therapy used by psychologists today. It has been effective for many people, but there are also setbacks with this type of therapy. CBT requires you to actively attempt to retrain the way you think.

In therapy and on your own, you are asked to record your negative thought. What was the situation that caused this negative thought? How did you react? What are five or more ways, you could have reacted better? The idea is that if you face the same situation again, you are able to think of a more positive response and use it. It is also a therapy, where you are asked to slow down and assess the situation.

If you stop, think, listen, correct your internal reaction, then you are able to gain a better overall reaction in various situations. Let's assess an example.

Say you are at work. You made a mistake. You are in a depressive state. You call yourself stupid, you say it aloud to others, and you are unhappy the rest of the day.

In therapy, you would be asked to stop, think about those thoughts, and listen to how harmful they are.

You would then need to determine how you could have reacted better, such as saying "I made a mistake. It does not make me less of a person, but I do need to learn from this mistake, and try to avoid it in the future."

In this way, you acknowledge the problem, you accept that mistakes happen because people are not perfect, and you will learn from it in the future.

Therapy can also be one-on-one sessions, where you talk about your feelings. Sometimes you just need to talk, to unload, and you are able to see things clearly. It is not complaining or useless time, as long as the person helping you works with depression. You want someone who is an expert in depression versus a common therapist or counselor, particularly if you have severe depression.

Support Groups

Support groups should be used in conjunction with therapy. Support groups provide you with a place to go and talk about your troubles, with others who share the same troubles. Seeing that others are in difficult situations and depressed can help you reflect on your own behavior.

Changing Relationships

Not all relationships are healthy for you. Some relationships enable you to continue being depressed. Other relationships are not giving you what you need, such as support and attention. Changing these relationships can help you find your self-worth and get on the path to recovery.

Herbal Remedies

St. John's Wart is just one herb known to help with depression on a short-term basis. There are also teas with herbs in them that are known to help with depression because they help calm you and correct hormonal imbalances. Herbs are not always the answer and should not be taken unless you speak with a physician or mental health professional first.

Chapter 8: New Approaches and Methods to Treat Depression

Researchers are consistently looking for ways to treat depression. There is not a specific cure all for depression. Some treatments work for certain patients, but not to others. To a degree, researchers are still asking questions about why depression occurs. Yes, there are certainly specific causes depression has been linked to; however, there some individuals that find no help in current treatments.

There are still unanswered questions about the hereditary properties of depression in certain family groups. All of these unanswered questions are leading researchers towards new methods of treatment, with the aim of treating more patients successfully.

One new approach to depression has targeted brain dysfunctions, cognitive, and emotional processes, which trigger depression symptoms. Greg J. Siegle is the director of the Program in Cognitive Affective Neuroscience, located at the University of Pittsburgh School of Medicine. Dr. Siegle states their new approach is to think of the brain as a muscle, which has atrophied, like the heart muscle atrophies during a stroke. He believes the brain is a muscle that needs to be rehabbed.

Their efforts have been to study the effects of computer games, math problems, and audio chirping birds to stimulate the emotional regulation of the brain. Other researchers use words and faces to help depressed individuals to disengage from the negative stimuli and focus on positive stimuli.

Computer games are used along with electrical stimulation of the brain in some studies. These treatments have mixed results. Scientists are working to determine the appropriate doses and they know that this therapy protocol will not work for all patients. The concept behind the new approach is to try something for individuals that have certain brain dysfunction leading to depression.

Scientists have taken images of depressed brains to try to map the areas of the brain affected by the disorder. They are working on treatments that target these areas in an attempt to "heal" the brain (Petersen, 2015).

Cognitive Control Training

Dr. Siegle is just one of the professionals working on depression treatments, who believe old therapies are not offering the greatest help possible. Simon Rego is the director of psychology training located at the Montefiore Medical Center in New York. Dr. Rego believes cognitive behavioral therapy or CBT is too hard for people suffering from depression. CBT is a retraining of the brain to stop thinking negatively, by analyzing the situation, your reaction, and coming up with positive ways to assess the emotions.

Dr. Rego feels people who are depressed have low energy, motivation, and concentration. It is difficult for a therapy to ask for a task to be completed that is opposite of what one's energy level is.

CCT is his alternative suggestion. With Cognitive Control Training, a person suffering from depression is asked to perform two exercises that last 15 minutes each. The patients are given numbers that are in a series. These numbers have set rules. The task is an attempt to activate an area of the prefrontal cortex called the dorsal lateral. It is the part of the brain associated with emotion regulation, as well as executive control. Dr. Siegle states it is an area that "voluntarily thinks" about something when you want it to. Dr. Siegle is part of the team that has developed CCT. He believes this underactive area of the brain is why many people ruminate on negative thoughts, which plague them, and make them feel depressed.

CCT includes listening to the sounds of birds chirping. These external sounds culminated with active and direct attention on the sounds, allows a person to concentrate on something other than their own thoughts.

The report, published in Behavioral and Cognitive Psychotherapy discussed a study that involved 48 people. These people suffered from depression. They were given three sessions of CCT. These sessions occurred in a two-week period. The depression scores dropped more significantly, than people obtaining CBT control exercises. The study was published in 2014.

A group located in Australia has also examined CCT with trans cranial direct current stimulation (tDCS). An electric current, on a gentle setting, is used while video games are played. A study called Brain Stimulation was published in 2014 based on this study. It showed depressed patients who had a combination of CCT and electrical stimulation experienced a 46% reduction in their symptoms after three weeks of treatment. Individuals who received only CCT saw a decrease in symptoms of only 17% and those with electrical stimulation only saw an 8.9% reduction.

Among the new therapies developed, Dr. Siegle has worked on exercises in concentration. He uses two electrodes on the arm, passing a very weak current through the body. The placement of the electrode causes an itching sensation that is extremely annoying. Patients find it difficult to think negative thoughts with this itching occurring (Petersen, 2015).

Interpretation Bias Modification

Interpretation Bias Modification is also called Cognitive Bias Modification-Interpretation (CBM-I). It is a new treatment Dr. Jamie Micco, at Harvard Medical School has been working on. Micco is an assistant professor. He stated CBM-I tries to contradict the way people look at ambiguous situations and then react negatively.

In one study, he had patients look at written scenarios. These scenarios were positively resolved, but often the last word was missing a letter and patients needed to fill it in. CBM-I's goal is to help patients think in a positive or neutral way, versus the negative their brain's focus on.

Further testing for CBM-I treatment has people look at two faces, one neutral in expression and the other sad. The patient is trained to look away from the negative and focus on the neutral, just as the patient is asked to focus on neutral words versus negative words.

The Journal of Abnormal Psychology published a study in 2015 relating to CBM as a way to reduce negative focus. The treatment contained a placebo, where 52 subjects were studied for four weeks. Patients noticed a 40% reduction in symptoms. The study's authors thought the placebo treatment actually enhanced the attention of patients, which helped reduce the symptoms patients felt.

The new approaches discussed focus mainly on the negative attention depressed patients have. They are biased towards negative thoughts versus positive thoughts. About 2/3 thirds of patients with depression have these rumination troubles, and the other third do not. It is very important for a trained professional to treat a patient with depression based on their symptoms, reactions to situations, and physical well-being. To be successful one has to understand the neurobiological and cognitive issue in the patient, so that treatment can be designed specifically for the patient (Petersen, 2015).

Treatment-Resistant Depression Approaches

Neuromodulation is one type of treatment patients are incorporating into their depression treatment, when all other methods have failed. It is designed to pass electrical current through the brain.

There are a couple of types of this treatment: electroconvulsive therapy, Vagus nerve stimulation and repetitive transcranial magnetic stimulation. These all use a type of weak electrical current that is transmitted by the electrodes. They work on stimulating specific areas of the brain, such as the Vagus nerve (University of Michigan, 2016).

The Vagus nerve supplies the lungs, heart, upper digestive tract and other organs. It is a cranial nerve that provides parasympathetic control of these organs. Research studies indicate stimulating these organs and the nerve can relieve pain, but also help a person retrain their brain to think in a more positive manner. It is also a nerve that Psychology Today links with "gut instincts."

A study in Switzerland found the nerve provides feelings, what we call gut instincts to the brain. These are the instinctual feelings that tell us when there is danger or when we have the right answer. By using electrical current, the nerve is stimulated to feel less "threatening" feelings, thus allowing happier thoughts to enter the brain.

This and the other treatments discussed are in early testing. Only small groups of people have been tested. As new approaches, these treatments are seemingly positive for certain types of patients.

If you have tried other treatments, without success or feel that CBT is too much work for your current depressive state, you may wish to find a study near you or ask your current physician/therapist about these options.

The more information you gather about potential help with your depression, the more comfortable and in control you will start to feel. Depending on the

However, it was clearly happening. Again, going to the physician she asked if, other than her thyroid troubles, something might have changed with her hormones. Again, the physician did not provide a proper reply. Armed with information that St. John's Wart, when used in limited quantities, could help with depression, she asked if she could start taking it. The idea was to take the herbal medicine a week or two prior to her period start date and see if there was an improvement.

After four months, she discovered a significant improvement. Taking a pill on a daily basis for a week prior to her period, this young woman had an easier time during the PMS stage. Her body also returned to normal, with fewer depressive episodes and she was able to track that every other month she suffered from worse PMS symptoms, with significant depression.

You may have to take the initiative in your health care and mental care. While physicians should be relied on for their expert medical knowledge, you may have to change how you approach your own care.

The example is not about the woman seeking her own medical advice online, but about reading information, so she was better armed to speak with her physician about her symptoms.

It is also about what else you can change. Feeling depressed, dealing with a busy life, and money concerns, she was unable to take action to find a new physician that might have heard her concerns with a better "bedside manner."

The experience has taught this person that if the physician is not going to learn, then it is paramount to her overall well-being to seek a new general practitioner. Your care is in your hands. You ultimately decide if you are going to follow a care plan, but you also have to have a physician who is willing to listen, take you seriously, and see your intelligence.

Depression is all about feeling unintelligent and worthless. You don't need a physician who is not going to listen or search for the underlying cause of your feelings. Rather, you need a person who will listen, who will refer you to the right people, and the person who is willing to help you.

You are the most important person in your care plan. You are the person who has to make changes to your situation to alleviate the turmoil you feel. When you are ready to accept these needs, you are ready to find a treatment plan that will work for you. Only when you are ready to seek help are you truly going to get the help you need. It comes from within you, as well as from the resources you have at your disposal.

Chapter 10: How to Find Fulfillment in Life

You can begin your own treatment. If you have sought a diagnosis from a physician or psychologist, you can work towards a treatment plan with them, as well as with yourself. Depression has many causes, but among them and often the most prevalent is feeling worthless, stupid, and low self-esteem. This cycle of emotions can be broken. These steps may not work for everyone. You may have tried them and found no success, but perhaps it was your self-discipline and approach.

The Mind is a Powerful Organ

Your mind is extremely powerful. It is the epicenter of your entire life. Without your brain, you would be an empty shell. The phrase "you cannot teach an old dog new tricks," is a myth. Worse, it is wrong. You can teach your aging brain new tricks. You can change how it reacts, thinks, and processes information. All you need to do is be willing and discover any underlying factors that might hinder this process.

Here are some things that may make these steps difficult:

- You have an illness, you do not know about, thyroid disorder, beginnings of dementia, or other hormonal imbalance.

- You suffer from a chemical imbalance.

- Your brain may not be connected properly via the nervous system.

- Genetic causes might be affecting your brain process.

- You are in the middle of a great loss, which is making your depression worse.

- You have PTSD (post-traumatic stress disorder) that is leading to depression.

Make absolutely certain that your depression is not a result of a biological condition. Also, assess the rest of your life to determine if PTSD, abuse, or a death in your immediate family/friends circle is making your depression worse. Armed with the best list of causes for your depression, means you are armed to correct all aspects of the depression, as well as gain fulfillment from life.

Your Treatment Plan

Beginning with the understanding of your depressions cause, you can now work on a self-treatment plan to find joy in life.

1. Get a journal or start one on your computer.

2. Keep this journal with you at all times.

3. On the first page, write out 1 positive feeling about yourself. It may be that you love your hair color, its length, or your eyes. You might write that you love the strength you have in difficult situations. No matter what it is, it needs to be a compliment.

4. Underneath this compliment, write 1 goal for your life. This goal can be obtaining a new job, going back to school, finishing school, travelling somewhere. The only caveat is the goal has to be something you can accomplish, realistically.

5. If it is a goal, such as going back to school, then your job is to take small steps towards this

long term goal. It can also be a short term goal. You might set a goal about waking up, lying in bed for 10 minutes, and thinking only of positive thoughts. Whatever goal you set, you need to be able to make it.

6. The next task is to create a meaning of life chart, diagram, map, or list. This is not about goals. It is about what would make life more meaningful to you. The Buddhists believe that the end to suffering is to forgo the materialistic things and desires we have. If you desire love and you have been unable to attain it, then you may feel depressed. So what are the things that have greater meaning?

How to see the Greater Meaning

When in the throes of depression, it is difficult, nearly impossible to see the greater meaning to your life. You tend to feel worthless versus meaningful. However, all is not lost.

Writing out your emotions is the best way to find what is most meaningful to you. A person lost her father. Her father was a friend and a mentor, as well as a loved one.

Instead, of being sad and angry at the loss, she focused on the meaning he gave to her life, the happy moments that they shared together. She did not forget about the times when they argued when she was growing up, but instead, remembered the lessons from those times.

She also had the most important lesson he gave to her and that was, "I have lived my life with no regrets." Her father taught her that all mistakes, disappointments, and happiness in life is where the meaning of life comes from. It is not about dwelling on the bad, on the things that cannot be changed, but the focus should be on the positive that was gained from any situation.

Those words held more power in getting over her depression and sense of loss than any others. Perhaps they can for you as well. Take time now to consider what has happened in your life that was good.

Was there a time you felt worthwhile? Was there a person who made you feel worthy and important? If you can find one happy memory, then you can start to recall the others. From this, you can discover true meaning in your life.

Most of us do not want to feel like our existence is for naught. Yet, we also know that life ends. You are born, you live, and you die. In death, the only thing that could bring meaning to your life is how you are remembered. For some, it is about accomplishing great feats—perhaps writing the great American novel. For others, it is the family they have, the lessons they have left behind, and the community influence they have provided.

You are not going to find the meaning in your life immediately. It can take a week, a month, a year, or several years. The point is not rushing to a solution about your depression and finding fulfillment immediately, but about the trip it takes you to get there. It is also about the changes you make, so you can get to a point of realizing what fulfillment truly means.

Conclusion

Thank you again for purchasing this book!

I hope this book was able to help you with your needs and to satisfy your reading pleasures.

Depression might have been misunderstood in the beginning, and we may not fully understand the disorder now. However, we are gaining more ground in our research around the world to start helping us find better treatment opportunities.

There is a cure for you. It may be a long road, with setbacks. If you are willing to take a journey to find more meaning in your life, then you will start to find a treatment plan that fits your needs.

You do have to admit to needing help, seek a professional who can help you, and you will start to feel better about yourself. Take the next step and start feeling better.

Finally, if you enjoyed this book, please take the time to share your thoughts and post a review on Amazon. It would be greatly appreciated!

Thank you and good luck!

References

Hall, A. (2014, September 03). *10 Depression Myths We need to Stop Believing*. Retrieved from Huffington Post: http://www.huffingtonpost.com/2014/09/03/depression-myths_n_5715453.html

Medicine Net. (n.d.). *Causes of Depression*. Retrieved from Medicine Net: http://www.medicinenet.com/script/main/art.asp?articlekey=55167

Petersen, A. (2015, June 1). *To Treat Depression, a new Approach Tries Training the Brain*. Retrieved from WSJ: http://www.wsj.com/articles/to-treat-depression-a-new-approach-tries-training-the-brain-1433178996

Reiss, N. (2007, September 19). *Historical Understandings of Depression*. Retrieved from Mental Help: https://www.mentalhelp.net/articles/historical-understandings-of-depression/

University of Michigan. (2016). *Three Minute Tips New Approaches for Treating Depression*. Retrieved from Psych Med U of Michigan: http://www.psych.med.umich.edu/expert-advice/treating-depression/

Webmd. (n.d.). *Depression Health Center*. Retrieved from Web MD: http://www.webmd.com/depression/guide/detecting-depression

Wikipedia. (2016, May 27). *History of Depression.* Retrieved from Wikipedia: https://en.wikipedia.org/wiki/History_of_depression#20th_and_21st_centuries

World Health Organization. (2016, April). *Depression Fact Sheet.* Retrieved from WHO: http://www.who.int/mediacentre/factsheets/fs369/en/

How to Analyze People: Using Human Psychology to Successfully Understand Anyone from Anyplace and Anywhere

Enhance your Social Skills, People Skills, Body Language, Relationships, Communication, Personality, and Nonverbal Cues

By Sammy Parker

Table of Contents

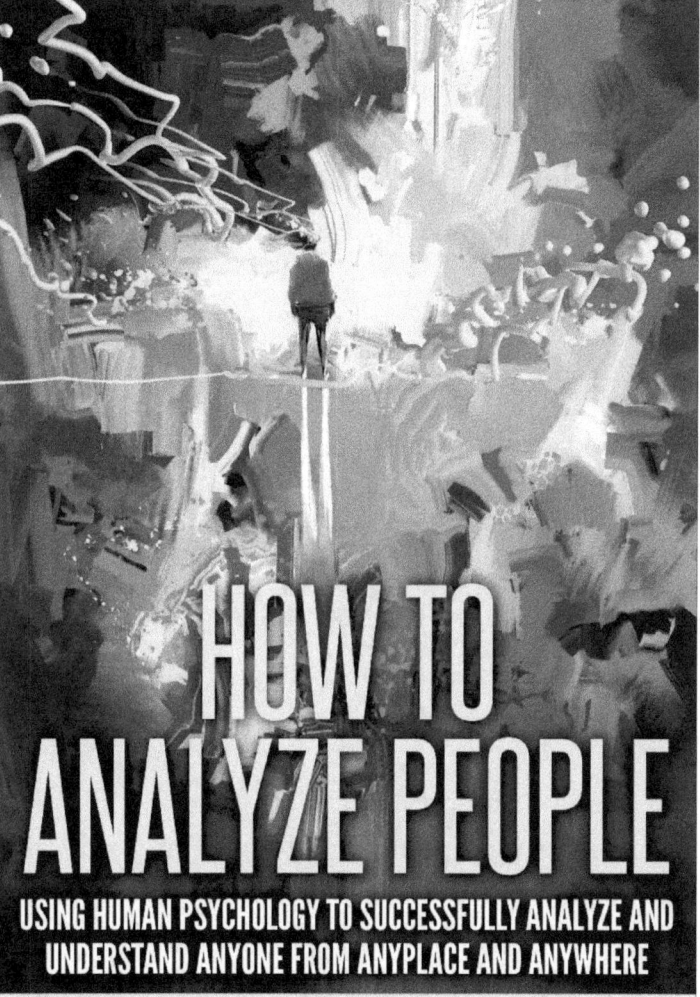

HOW TO
ANALYZE PEOPLE

USING HUMAN PSYCHOLOGY TO SUCCESSFULLY ANALYZE AND UNDERSTAND ANYONE FROM ANYPLACE AND ANYWHERE

Enhance your social skills, people skills, body language,
relationships, communication, personality, and nonverbal cues

SAMMY PARKER

Introduction

I want to thank you and congratulate you for downloading the book, *"How to Analyze People and Use Psychology to Understand Anyone"*.

This book contains proven steps and strategies on how to get better at picking up the signals others are sending you, both in words and in nonverbal cues, to improve your interactions with people, in general.

This is an important topic because this type of communication is happening constantly, whether we are aware of it or not. It runs our interactions and rules our social lives, often without us even realizing it. Becoming aware of this aspect of existence will open up new doors to improving our relationships and ourselves with people, whether it be acquaintances or close friends and relatives.

In this Book, you will learn:

- **How to get a Better Idea of What People are Trying to Tell you:** People are not always upfront about their thoughts, feelings, and intentions. In fact, most of the time, they are portraying a lot of these at once without even knowing it. The people who have the highest success rates in dating, friendships, and any other area of life that involves human interaction, are aware of this hidden communication and how to use it to propel themselves forward. We will cover this topic in a later chapter.

- **How to Become more Charismatic:** It can be hard to know exactly what to say, especially when it comes to people you don't know very well or just met. For this reason, a lot of people struggle with having a lack of charisma, which hinders them in countless aspects of life. In this book, you will learn some proven ways to become more charismatic and draw people to you.

- **How to Talk to Strangers more Easily:**
  Talking to strangers is difficult when you aren't
  aware that you possess a high level of charisma
  and ability to read the body language of others.
  Meeting people you don't know will come
  naturally to you after you read the facts and
  strategies outlined in this book.

- **How to be a Better Communicator:** It's
  happened to all of us more than once. We have
  a message we feel is important to get across, we
  try to communicate it to someone near us, and
  they completely misinterpret what we said and
  it causes a huge confusion and sometimes
  arguments. This is often due to having inferior
  communication skills. After reading this book,
  this is a situation that will happen to you less
  and less frequently.

In essence, what you're about to read is a guide to
yourself and others. You will find that the more you

understand about your own motivations, fears, and abilities to communicate, the more you will be able to read and interact with other people. The two go hand in hand, and this guide will help you with both.

Thanks again for downloading this book, I hope you enjoy it!

Chapter 1: How Knowing Body Language Helps You

We have all been in situations where we were either misunderstood by another person, misunderstood someone else, or even worse, a combination of the two. Some people are not very good at talking to strangers, making friends, or keeping existing relationships. A lot of these interpersonal misfortunes can be traced back to one very simple thing; being unaware of how to analyze others. This can lead to many headaches and rifts between others and us that do not have to be there. Luckily, there's hope for this.

Knowing how to Analyze Body Language will Help with:

- **Reading what is not Spoken:** Words are only a small portion of communication, and the rest comes across in our unspoken movements and gestures. Knowing how to analyze people will mean that you don't miss most of what is being communicated and know how to pay attention to it. This will help you become a master of communication.

- **Getting Messages Across more Clearly:** Once you understand how to read the unspoken cues of other people, you will better understand how to present yourself in ways that get across what you are trying to say. The people who are misinterpreted most often are usually not very aware of what their body language is saying. Sometimes, we say the exact opposite of what we mean or feel with our facial expressions or posture. Being aware of this side of things will make our thoughts and actions align.

- **Preventing Misunderstandings:** Being oblivious to the thoughts and feelings of others means that people see us as uncaring or perhaps even ignorant. This does not foster a healthy environment for healthy interactions or beneficial relationships. Taking it upon ourselves to learn about how to analyze the behavior of others and how to present ourselves more accurately means that communication, as a whole, becomes easier and we are presented with better opportunities throughout life.

These are just a few of the ways that body language can help you. It will also help you become more charismatic, since you will be more aware of your expressions than ever. Charisma is an important aspect of human life.

How Having Charisma Helps you with Life:

- **People Trust you More:** If you're a charismatic person, people tend to like you a lot more and a lot more often. This increases their level of trust in you meaning that they see you as someone they can rely on. This helps in personal situations as well as professional events or even interacting with people you have never met before. When you are a likeable person, doors open up where they never were before.

  Old relationships can blossom in entirely new ways, you will find strangers opening up to you with an ease they never had before, and you will find it much easier to connect with people you just met, increasing opportunities.

- **It Helps you Stand Out Professionally:**
  The job market can be a competitive place,
  especially when you know that 10 other people
  are applying the same job as you. So, how do
  you stand out at an interview? By having
  unbeatable charisma. Work places get more
  and more competitive as time goes on, and the
  only way to stay relevant and up to date is to
  make sure that your personality is top notch.

  This is a must if you want to gain great
  professional positions, keep the jobs, and also
  advance far in your professional life. This goes
  hand in hand with the trust that being
  charismatic brings, since bosses are more likely
  to promote people they trust.

- **Making Friends is Easier:** Having friends,
  especially a wide assortment of them, improves
  life vastly. Not only will you have access to
  more differing perspectives, interests, and
  hobbies, but you are opened up to a whole new
  world of personalities that you can look to for
  improving your own. You will also be better
  connected, meaning you have more people to
  rely on or to help you in hard times or with
  favors.

  When you have a large friend group, you have a
  person to talk to about anything, no matter
  what subject arises, because of all of the
  different people you know and trust. This can

only be possible when you are well aware of the body language of yourself and others.

Everyone wishes to be an intelligent and likeable person with a lot of influence. The only way this is possible is through knowing how to accurately read what others are trying to say and by getting a handle on the way we come across to others.

Chapter 2: How to Improve Communication

Now that we have identified the reasons why being aware of body language in ourselves and others is so important, we can get down to the basics of conversation. This isn't something that comes naturally to everyone, and most of us have to practice a lot before we become great at it. So, if you're starting out with getting comfortable talking to others, where do you begin?

- **Meet as Many People as Possible:** This can be a tough one, especially for people who are shy, but how can you improve your speaking abilities if you don't interact with many people? The first and most crucial step to being better at analyzing others and communicating with them effectively is putting yourself in more situations where you are interacting with new people. Over time, you will get better and better at reading their gestures, because being around other individuals will become so comfortable and natural. This may be hard at first, and you may find yourself distracted or overwhelmed by your surroundings, but this will improve the more you do it.

- **Don't be Afraid to Ask for Clarification:** Misunderstandings often happen because people are too shy to double check on something that someone said or did, and instead make assumptions. This habit helps no one and only treats tension where it doesn't have to exist. Whether you are talking to someone you know well and love, or a new person, if you aren't entirely sure what they meant by something they said, don't hesitate to ask! People are often more receptive to frank honesty than we think they will be, and showing this very human side of you creates rapport.

- **Get Feedback from Loved and Trusted Sources:** It's easy to see the qualities of others, but hard to see our own. For this reason, valuable insight can be gained from asking those close to us about our own traits that might be invisible or hard to see ourselves. Ask the three people around you who spend the most time with you on a daily basis what your great qualities are, and what aspects of yourself can use some work.

This will help you not only be more open and humble to the opinions of others, but learn how to improve your personality, which will bring you countless benefits in life. Don't forget to stay open for this exercise and remember not to get offended easily. If you think that a person you are asking would try to offend you with their answers, you should ask another source.

- **Start a Journal:** Becoming great at communicating with others starts in the way we talk to ourselves. Since many of us don't walk around having conversations aloud with ourselves, it can be hard to know exactly what those conversations look like. In fact, many times, they are subconscious and we know nothing about them!

  The best way to get around this is to start a journal and write in it every single day. Even if you don't know what to say at first, you will figure it out quickly. This offers you a peek into the stream of your own mind, and once you get to know your own thoughts better, you will become better with interacting with others. This is because, when becoming aware of our own stream of thoughts, they cannot distract us as much when we interact with other people. This is one problem that occurs a lot and gets in the way of communication.

- **Talk to Strangers more Often:** What is the best way to get better at talking to people? By talking to people, of course. You may be telling yourself that you "don't know how" or feel intimidated at the prospect, if you're the shy type, but this is one surefire way to get great at it.

If you aren't used to this, it may be a bit scary at first, but you will quickly learn that people are nothing to fear and are often a lot nicer than we think they would be. The more you practice speaking around strangers, the more comfortable you will become and you will eventually wonder why you held back from it for so long.

- **Join an Internet Forum:** This may sound like the opposite of communication to some, but starting conversations (and often, friendships) online is a great way to improve your speaking and ability to articulate your thoughts. No matter what your interest is, there is probably a forum for it, filled with people who are just as excited as you are about the subject.

This is a great way to get conversation flowing naturally with people you don't know. Here, you will encounter new questions and ideas, and in formulating your answers, you will discover that your ability to express yourself gets stronger and stronger, and not just on the internet.

- **Get Over the Fear of Looking like a Fool:** One of the biggest reasons we either hold back from talking to others or we filter ourselves in conversation is that we are afraid of how we will look to others. Where we are going wrong with this line of reasoning is that this type of withholding and hesitation is what creates the awkward tension that we all fear and try to avoid so much.

People who have been influential or seen as cool or confident people are always the ones who don't worry too much about what others think. This gives them a confident aura that others are inspired from, since it is quite rare. Keep in mind that everyone feels insecure sometimes and that there is nothing wrong with being nervous. Even when you are afraid, make yourself get out there and talk to people anyway.

Chapter 3: Building up your Charisma

It seems, at times, like charisma is something that you are either born with or not, but all people are actually capable of creating and improving their own charisma. Regardless of what your personality is like now, there are specific qualities you can become aware of and use with your behaviors that will likely make you more influential, trustworthy, and all around likeable. Here is some basic information about how to build up your charisma.

It's Learned, not Inherent in Humans:

When we meet someone we like, we can rarely explain exactly what it is about him or her that draws us in so much. This means that they possess charisma. You can also learn how to be charismatic, and it's easier than you may think. It involves a few small changes to the way you behave. This quality is all about the things you say and the actions you partake in, rather than your deeper qualities. Your nonverbal cues, subconscious attitudes, physical motions, and the respect you have for other people are all involved with your level or charisma and the steps you will take to improve it.

Although this is a simple process, it does take some bravery on your part. Building up your charisma is an event that will require a close look at your actions. This often leads to seeing things you don't particularly like, but it's important not to get hung up on that, since it happens to everyone who becomes self-aware.

If you know how to check your expectations instead of getting stuck on them, you will be able to see which behaviors of yours need to be changed. Keep in mind that you don't need to fundamentally change everything about your core self, only the way those around you will perceive you by tweaking your outward expressions. Here are some real, actionable steps for gaining and keeping charisma:

Learn how to be Present:

This is one of, if not the most crucial factor in building charisma, along with knowing how to exude confidence. Being present means that you know how to engage with other people in a real way. In essence, you are showing the individual you are interacting with that they have your focus.

- **Be Aware of How you Come Across to Other People:** When someone isn't confident, they can often come across as someone who doesn't have any interest in other people, even when the opposite is true. Without knowing how to be present for others in conversation, you could come across as arrogant or uncaring. Neither of these extremes is something to hope for. Being present for others shows them that they are worth your time and that you care to hear them out. Nothing works better for building respect and trust than this.

- **It's about Helping Others Feel Good about Themselves:** Some people may think of charisma and automatically have ideas of seeming awesome and confident in the eyes of other people, but the true secret to it involves more than this. Charisma is not about showcasing your greatness to the world, but about knowing how to make another feel great about them. This means that they feel important, worthwhile, and leave a conversation with you feeling better about life and their own worth than they did prior to the interaction.

- **Know What People Like to Discuss:** An inescapable fact about humans is that we enjoy speaking about the subject we are most familiar with; ourselves. When you like someone or find them charismatic or magnetic, it's usually because they allow you to talk about your interests and be yourself. Stay optimistic, turn your ego off, and be present for people when they are speaking to you. It can truly be as simple as this.

- **Find Ways to Stay Intrigued and Focused:** Give your utmost focus to everything that the other is saying, imagining that you are focusing on a book or movie and that they are the most important character, if this helps you. A lot of people talk to others while just focusing on what they are going to say next, without truly listening. This comes across in interactions and is a huge turnoff. While this may seem like you are truly engaging in the conversation, you aren't, and it doesn't seem as though you are listening when you do this.

Of course, this involves a balance of listening and speaking. It's not good to simply sit and be a listening ear for everyone without getting the same favor in return. Being aware of how to express yourself and speak to others in a way that exudes confidence is equally important to listening.

Increase your Level of Personal Confidence:

Learning how to become confident will give you a gigantic advantage when you decide to undertake the journey to developing charisma, but this is easier said than done. If it were as simple as deciding to have confidence, everyone would do it, and it wouldn't even be a noteworthy quality. You shouldn't want to come across as arrogant or self-absorbed, but it's equally negative to seem scared or timid in social situations. What it all relies on is your own level of comfort with yourself.

- **Confidence begins with the Physical**
  Staying active and in shape, wearing items that make you feel nice about yourself, and focusing on conversation topics that you can contribute to will make you feel more confident about yourself.

- **Don't Fear not Knowing about Certain Topics:** This doesn't mean that you should only speak about things you are an expert in, however. It's perfectly possible to stay on an open level with people and show them that you are interested and curious while still staying confident and assertive. A lot of people get frozen up when we find ourselves in a talk that we aren't knowledgeable about, which makes us defensive and oftentimes, awkward. We may shift to a position of trying to hide our own lack of knowledge, when simply being comfortable with our ignorance would come across as way more likeable and relatable to others.

- **Maintain an Open and Curious Demeanor:** If you learn how to switch, at will, from this mode of defense to a mode of openness and curiosity, you will come across as a confident person who is okay with the fact that they aren't knowledgeable about a certain subject. In addition to this, staying in a curious frame of mind will help you stay present, which we mentioned the importance of earlier. You won't be tuning out of the conversation or rehearsing what you will say next, you will seem truly present for the other person.

- **Find a Reason to Live:** When someone has charisma and confidence, their lives have a purpose. Not having a driving force or mission in life is something that is visible and noticeable to others, and it isn't a very attractive quality to be missing this essential characteristic. This doesn't mean that you have to enthusiastically rave about your passion at every chance you get, but you must be aware of and confident about the fact that you are alive for a reason.

- **Focus your Energies:** Select a goal, cause, or vision to become passionate about and life. Most individuals go through life searching for a reason to live or a cause to truly put their faith in. You must embody your passion so intensely that it is noticeable to others.

- **Fake it till you Make it:** Believe in yourself in every situation and show that you are not bothered by the doubts that overtake most others. Pretend like you know where you are going and why, even if you aren't completely certain. This helps a lot with developing confidence, over time. Even when you aren't sure where you are headed, you should appear to be aware.

- **Pretend it's a Movie:** As soon as a certain scenario starts playing out, pretend to be aware of exactly what your next lines are.

- **Forget Mistakes as Soon as Possible:** Everyone has times when we say or do something and feel, later, that it was the dumb thing to say or do. Do yourself a favor and banish those moments from your memory. When those situations occur and you stop to ruminate on what just happened, the way you appear to others changes immediately. You start to hesitate and others can notice this.

Being confident means that you are okay with what type of person you are and the things you do, regardless of what this specifically entails. People are drawn to people who have confidence, regardless of what their other traits are like. Once you master the art of confidence, charisma is the next logical step.

Learn Conversation Basics:

People who have charisma are good at talking to others. They are aware of the best ways to begin conversations, keep them interesting, and hold the attention of others, always making them feel comfortable. If you aren't aware of how to communicate with those around you, it's an inescapable fact that you must practice this. Sure, it won't be easy, at first, but being brave and getting away from the self-doubting personality traits will hold many benefits, in the end.

- **Learn to Stop Avoiding Discomfort:** Most people avoid uncomfortable situations like the plague, which is why charismatic people, who aren't paralyzed by the fear of looking stupid or saying the wrong thing, stand out so much. Get over the fear of uncomfortable situations and put yourself out there to develop charisma.

  If you are unaware of how to begin conversations, don't be afraid to use your creativity to come up with ideas. Firstly, you can muse to yourself about which topic you would prefer to discuss and which you would not. If it so happens that there are topics that you want to avoid, it's probably safe to assume that many others would as well. Keep in mind that it's usually simpler and easier to start a conversation by simply being nice instead of trying to come across as smart.

- **Opt for Nice rather than Impressive:** Trying to seem impressive or highly intelligent can either come across as bragging or arrogant, or just intimidate others, which does nothing to improve charisma. In addition to this, being nice to others is one of the quickest ways to instantly boost your charisma levels. If you are having trouble thinking of a way to open a conversation or find yourself in a lull during the talk, just find a way to avoid silences that could be awkward. More often than not, people will appreciate the effort.

- **Meet People on the Same Level:** People who are great at conversation know exactly how to get others on their level. They do this by sharing personal stories or telling about experiences in their life that relate to what others say. This has to be done in an artful way that doesn't attempt to shift the focus of the talk over to you, but only makes the other person feel understood and related to.

- **Rely on Humor, but in a Smart Way:** Charismatic people are often funny, but they know how to do it and when to hold off. Don't be afraid to use the valuable tool of humor but keep in mind that the way you say things is often more important than what you are saying. If you are uncertain about whether a joke is appropriate, it's best to hold back. No one will even know about it and it's much safer than risking an awkward moment.

- **Be Interested Enough in Others to Ask them About Themselves:** Everyone wants ot feel as though they are being heard, and the best way to give them this feeling is to ask them interested questions. The individual who leads the inquiries is usually at the head of the business meeting. People who come up with intelligent questions always come across as smart, which improves their level or perceived charisma to other people around them.

While many people focus a lot on how their answers will come across, charisma often lies in the ability to know how to ask questions. Asking questions doesn't require special knowledge the way giving quality answers does, but the ones who ask the right questions are often the most likeable of all.

For an example of this phenomenon, envision the host of your favorite talk show. They are likely a very charismatic person, which is how they landed that job. Although they are so charming and likeable, they are usually doing nothing but inquiring about their guests, and come across as in control and highly likeable. Being charismatic has more to do with caring about others than it does coming across as knowledgeable or impressive.

Get Better at Holding Eye Contact with Others:

As mentioned earlier in the book, most of communication has nothing to do with words, and eye contact is a perfect example of this. Quality eye contact has the ability to communicate far more than speech does. It can show that you care about the person speaking, that you are taking the time to listen, and that you respect the other person's individuality and rights as a person. If you can't stop looking away of averting your gaze, it could come across that you are not interested in them, even if this isn't true.

- **Find the Right Amount be Experimenting:** This is a tricky subject because too much eye contact can have negative consequences, while too little is also bad. To get past this conundrum you can practice keeping your eye contact for just a bit longer, next time you're talking to someone. How does this shift the communication? How does it change how the other reacts or how you feel about the conversation?

Keep in mind that there are countless chances to practice this method, including people who live with you or strangers out in public that you interact with. You can even try it with your waiter or the person sitting across from you on the train.

- **Try to Remember People's Eye Colors:** Eventually, you will figure out what works for you with holding eye contact and what is unnecessary. The way you initiate eye contact is equally important as the length of time you hold the gaze. If you don't know where you should begin and are afraid of coming across as strange, attempt to focus on the other person's eye color.

Make it a point to pay attention to the color of everyone's eyes that you interact with and turn this into a regular habit. This will come across as friendly, interested eye contact rather than the dreaded creepy kind we all wish to avoid.

Don't Forget to Use your Body to Express Yourself:

Magnetic, charismatic personalities are expressive in a number of ways. When you know how to use your entire body to enhance what you're saying or emphasize your feelings, it does a lot to improve your quality of communication. Nobody finds stiff people interesting, magnetic, or charismatic.

- **Don't Forget to Smile:** People who smile are far more likeable and approachable than people who appear uninterested or angry. If often only takes a few seconds of holding a smile to begin to genuinely feel happy, then the rest comes without effort. Be someone that people feel comfortable approaching by smiling instead of appearing neutral or negative.

- **Observe Others First:** If you don't know where to begin with expressing yourself more often physically, you can begin by paying more attention to those around you, including animals. Think of the most physically expressive people you know who captivate an entire room with their gestures, or your pet dog when he gets excited to see you after a long day at work.

People like to be around others, as well as pets, who have a wide range or gestures that are highly expressive. This doesn't mean you need to be over the top with it or fake, but physical gestures that correspond with events that are happening and are relevant to the situation at hand are appealing and winning. They do a lot to increase your charisma.

- **Stay Aware of Negative Physical Expressions, too:** While focusing more on your physical gestures, it's important to be aware of what can come across as negative, in this regard. To take an example, nodding your head is a positive gesture to show a person that you are paying attention to what they are saying, but dong this too often can look awkward, wrong, and out of place. This can be a lot worse than not moving whatsoever.

Going over the top with your gestures can show to the other that you are attempting to come across a certain way and trying to make up for a lack of something. This means that they won't feel validated or safe around you anymore. Since individuals can sense your expressions, even the tiniest ones, learning to be aware of them is a great benefit to you.

If you are uncertain about what gestures you might do that come across as negative or awkward, you can ask a close and trusted loved one for advice. Remember that this might not be pleasant to hear, but you can never improve if you aren't aware of what areas you need to work on.

- **Stay Aware of your Gestures and Body Language:** Similar to actors learning to embody a character they are portraying, you should learn to get into a state of being that helps you stay conscious of how you are behaving. This can be something as simple as focusing on your breathing or simply feeling your body parts. Learn to realize when you are slouching or coming across in a negative way to others.

Learn how to Mirror Others in Conversation:

Humans are automatically drawn to others who have something in common with them, whether they are aware of it or not. Learning how to mirror the qualities of others is a quick and simple way to have charisma immediately. Make it a point to reflect back a person's level of energy or mannerisms and the effect it as will be noticeable right away.

- **It's not about Constantly Agreeing:** Mirroring doesn't mean you are trying to be exactly like the other person or need to agree with them on absolutely everything, but that you are meeting them on their level. With people who get along well or are great friends, this happens unconsciously, but it can be consciously engineered to increase charisma.

- **Emulate Charismatic Qualities in Other People:** Knowing how to observe and learn from others is a huge part of being charismatic. If you want to master this skill, the first place you should look is to people you find highly charismatic. This does not mean attempting to steal another person's personality or directly copying everything they do, but instead it means becoming aware of their secrets and what makes them great, testing them out for yourself and seeing what fits you.

- **Discover your Own Personal Methods:** The idea is experimenting plenty until you find the right methods that work for you, and this often involves borrowing methods from others that you respect. There is no "one size fits all" method, when it comes to anything. We can only look to experts and hope to learn from them by adjusting their ideas to our own lives and personalities until we find a good fit.

- **Observe Performers or Famous People:** You can find a lot of valuable tips on charisma by looking to Hollywood stars or anywhere else that you notice people with a lot of charisma. Pay attention to how they walk or speak. It's true that some of them might be arrogant or conceited, but this doesn't mean we can't learn from their charismatic or effective traits and use them for yourself. Learn how to borrow likeable traits from others and turn them into your own.

Everyone, including you, has the capability to become more charismatic and charming, meaning that others will like you more and more. The shifts you need to make and the adjustments that must be made for this to occur are not as huge or intimidating as you may think.

Simply become present for others, develop confidence, and work on mastering your physical gestures, over time, and observe the way others start reacting to you. Keep in mind that this pursuit, like any other worthwhile undertaking, will not happen instantly, but instead will be a process. As long as you are taking small steps in the right direction, each day, you are doing great!

Chapter 4: Meeting New Friends

Humans are social creatures, which means that having friends is valuable for everyone, no matter who they are or what their life situation is. They are the people we can turn to when things go bad, or celebrate with when things are great. It's hard to make friends or keep them if you don't know how to read body language or present yourself in the correct ways.

A very common problem that people have socially is that they are uncertain about how to make new friends or build a group of friends. This can be due to a variety of factors.

People Might have Difficulty with Friendships because:

- **They have Recently Moved and Haven't had a Chance to Socialize Yet:** This is perhaps the most familiar issue people face when moving to a new city. The reason moving can be so intimidating is because you are leaving everyone you know to start over, and building social groups doesn't come quickly or easily.

- **Their Friendships have Fallen by the Wayside due to a Serious Relationship:** This is a sadly common phenomenon. People forget about their friend groups because their romantic interest takes up most of their time or attention.

- **Old Friendships have Withered Naturally:** Another reason that people may have a lack of friends in life is because their old relationships have tapered off due to factors out of their control. This could be their friends moving to new cities, getting busy with their careers or starting families. An extreme version of this can happen when all friendships are concentrated in one area that is no longer there, such as a class ending and people all moving away at the same time.

- **Growing Apart from Old Friends and Wishing for New Ones:** Sometimes you simply grow out of friendships and would rather seek out relationships with new people who fit better with you. This can cause an awkward overlap where your social life is strangely empty.

- **Shifting from Preferring Solitude to Wishing for Friends:** People could feel a strong desire for friends in their life if they used to be the type who was a bit of a loner and have suddenly changed to someone who prefers to be around people and make friends.

- **Shyness or Fear of Speaking to People:** Obviously, a lack of friendships can result from someone being shy or not knowing how to approach others. Some people may be entirely unaware of how to talk to others and, as a result, have no social life.

- **Abrupt and Intense Life Changes:** When people make huge shifts in their habits or behavior, such as quitting drinking or even drastic eating habit changes, this can cause a shift in their social circle, since they may not fit in as well with their old one anymore.

Now that we have identified some of the common reasons people may be noticing a lack of friendships in their life, we will go over some methods for gaining new friendships. First we'll go over basics and then get into some more complex principles and attitudes that are crucial to the process of making friends. You will notice that people who seem to be natural at making new friends already do the stuff on the list.

How to Make New Friends:

Here are the easiest and simplest steps to building friendships. Some of them may seem obvious or simplistic, but each point can hold a lot of material. If you're someone who struggles with social life, in general, you might come across at least one of these.

- **Discover some Potential Friendships:** In order to find some new friends, you have to discover possibilities for who this could be. This can involve either looking to your existing contacts for potentials. Obviously, this doesn't work so well if you have just moved somewhere new and haven't met anyone yet, but usually people already have the makings of a friend group around them without even realizing it.

  This doesn't mean you have to force yourself to go out on the town and talk to every stranger you see. You may find it better to look to existing people in your life and depending bonds with them rather than starting completely from scratch in building friendships. There may even be a few people you know already who are great candidates.

This could be acquaintance you get along with but don't see often. People you work with or go to school with and have an easy time talking to. Friends of family members or acquaintances. This could also be people you used to know well and have fallen out of contact with. Looking for ways to get the most out of your existing connections can be very helpful, but sometimes it's not enough. At times, you may be in a position where it's necessary to find complete strangers as potential friends.

- **Put Yourself in Unfamiliar Situations:** Putting yourself into situations where lots of new people are surrounding you at all times, and it's more than likely that at least one of them will stand out to you as a potential friend. This involves places like classes or work places. If you meet just a couple of nice people and meet up with them and their circle of acquaintances, odds are you will find new friends quite quickly.

- **Join New Communities:** Getting into brand new hobbies or interests, as well as joining new communities, is a great way to meet a lot of new friends. This will start friendships based on common interests so that you naturally have topics to discuss and things in common. You can find these by searching online for groups in your town.

To start with, getting to know strangers may take some extra effort out of your natural, daily routine. If a lot of your interests take place alone, you should find ways to get interested in events that involve more people. In addition to this, the simplest way to get to know lots of people is to be an excited person who engages in plenty of new activities and draws others to them naturally as a result.

The More People you Talk to, the Better Odds you Have:

As soon as you find yourself living a life where you have a lot of potential friends around you, you can figure out ways to start conversations and get acquainted with them in a deeper way. This won't lead to forming lasting bonds every time you interact with someone new, but if you put yourself out there often and find ways to talk to plenty of people you are drawn to, it's bound to happen.

You will even find that you mesh quite well with a lot of them. As soon as you have done this, you can confidently say that you have moved from common acquaintances, to friends. If meeting people and talking to them doesn't come easily to you, you may want to do some extra research on overcoming shyness and insecurity.

Invite New People to do Activities with you:

As soon as you have come across potentially interesting friend candidates who you click well with, you can approach the and see if they would like to do something with you outside of the current situation you are both in. This is a crucial step, and it's what separates acquaintances from actual friends. You can meet countless people and get along great with them, but if you never go beyond that and broach the subject of hanging out with them outside of work or school, you will never form deeper bonds with anyone. This will mean that potential friends stay someone you chat with only at work or school. You could be missing out on great opportunities by not approaching these candidates.

This may seem simple and obvious, but people who are more solitary by nature and perhaps a bit lonely can hit a wall at this point. There could be a person that they feel comfortable joking with at their workplace or even enjoy chatting with in between classes at school, but they are unsure of how to take the next step. In order to form friendships, you must learn to be the one who steps outside of this acquaintance level to attempt to make friends.

This may be more Difficult for Shy People:

If you are a shy person, this might be difficult for you. Sure, it's a little unsettling the first few times you do it, and you are risking that they say no, but you can get used to this quite easily, and you have to if you want to make friends. The plus side to this is it's a lot easier to ask a potential friend to meet up outside of school or work than it is to ask someone out for a romantic outing.

How Long it Takes to Invite them Out Differs Depending on Situations:

It depends on how you met the person, but you may end up inviting them to hang out outside of school or work quite fast or even end up waiting a month or more. For example, if someone you know brings a friend of theirs to an outing you go on, and you had an easy time talking to them all night, it may be totally natural to ask them to meet up again right off the bat.

In another situation, if you seem to hit it off quite well with someone at work, it may be hard to tell whether it's just a professional courtesy to get along or whether there is real potential for friendship outside of the work place. This may mean that you only talk every once in a while and don't know how to approach the subject of inviting them out with you.

Here are some Examples of How to Invite Potential Friends Out:

- **Make it Normal and Natural to get People's Contact Info:** If you desire to make new friends, the best thing you can do for yourself is getting into a habit of asking for new people's contact information early on in meeting. It's possible you could meet someone cool or intriguing, but you can't know for sure that you are going to meet them again, and opportunities are often lost this way.

Get comfortable with asking for people's e-mail addresses, phone numbers, or social media profiles. This ill mean that if another chance comes up to meet, you can easily reach out to them. In addition to this, if they also have your information, they can reach out to you to invite you to events.

- **Figure out How to Instigate Plan-Making with Others:** To get to know a potential friend, which requires hanging out with them, you have to know how to plan for it. At times, this is a simple and straight forward process. You request someone to do something with you, they say yes, you come up with a place and a time, and you're done.

However, other times can be a bit more complicated, particularly when there are a lot of people involved. You can have difficulty deciding on a place to meet or a time that works for everyone. You can keep in mind that there is always uncertainty attached to these events and that not everything is within your control. Trying is all you can do, at times. If you find that asking people to come hang out with you and trying to arrange plans sounds like a huge inconvenience, remember that others probably feel the same. Take turns organizing events with the people you know.

- **Try to Accept Invitations to go Out with Others:** Organizing plans with acquaintances is necessary and crucial to making friends, but make sure that when others approach you and invite you somewhere, you take them up on the offer. When we get into certain patterns of spending a lot of time alone or becoming workaholics, it can be tempting to turn down people's attempts to get us out of the house, especially if you are shy. You may find yourself tempted to rationalize reasons to stay home, even though you've really been wishing for new friends lately. Don't accept these excuses and force yourself to go.

In fact, this situation is even better than inviting others out because you know for a fact that person is interested in getting to know you more. There's no good reason to turn down a chance to meet new people and make friends. Who knows what this could lead to?

At times, you may find that you have to go through something inconvenient to develop your social circle and meet new friends. Maybe you will get invited to a show you're not very interested in, or someone might give you a call on an evening when you were about to go to sleep. It's to be expected that you will have to compromise at times, especially when groups of people are involved in the process of planning events. Regardless of that, these situations should never be avoided.

You should also remember that if you say no to many times to people's invitations, they may stop asking altogether. So, get out there next time you're invited somewhere.

- **Remember to Stay in Touch and Keep the Relationship Going:** You may meet up with someone once or even twice and consider them beyond an acquaintance level after that. For certain, specific people, this may be enough to be considered a friend. However, if you're hoping to build lasting, meaningful connections that go beyond the surface, it's not enough to only meet up every once in a while.

The more you see each other in new circumstances and the more you experience together, the better potential there is for growing closer and building a strong bond. This shouldn't be expected to happen with every acquaintance you have, but if you continue making it a point to meet new people and explore friendship possibilities with them, it should be only a matter of time before you make some close friendships that can grow into possibly lifelong bonds.

Start with the Foundation of Knowing a Couple People:

As soon as you have made a friend, or a few, you have a great starting point to build up from. If you are not really the social type naturally, this may be all you require to feel fulfilled. If you were feeling sad and lonely before, it will do wonders for you to have a couple of people to hang out with. Eventually, you will find yourself meeting with friends of your friends. If it turns out that you get along well with them, your social circle just got even bigger! It's also possible that you could become a part of the entire circle of friends, over time.

There's also the possibility that you can pursue meeting others in addition to this. Once you have friends, this will get easier since it opens the door to more events, opportunities, and new people to meet.

Go through the Steps Above Repeatedly to Meet even More People:

If you end up joining a new organization and meet a few nice people there, go to hang out with one of them and meet some of their friends, you have just taken a huge step in the social realm. However, if you pause right here and stagnate, that's all you will have. If you keep at it and come up with new ways to meet potential friends constantly, eventually you will find yourself with a lot of friends to hang out with.

It all depends on your personality type. Some people can have an unlimited amount of friends and feel very happy about that, while others would feel overwhelmed going past a certain number. It's all about what you feel most comfortable with. Don't forget that you can always search for more if you end up feeling the urge to do so.

Other Basic Principles to Keep in Mind:

Now that we have gone over the basic elements to meeting new people and making friends, we can get into other concepts that apply to the situation. These are principles that need to be kept in mind when attempting to understand social dynamics and build lasting bonds with other people.

- **Your Social Circle is your Responsibility:** A basic principle to making a group of friends is taking the first initiative. Some people make the huge mistake of waiting around for others to take the initiative to befriend them, invite them to things, and pursue a connection with them beyond work or school. Sure, that may happen sometimes, which is great, but you should never expect that or depend on it.

  If you have made the decision that you want a social circle, come to terms with the fact that you need to make an effort to get it. If you are feeling active and desire to do something on Friday, don't just wait around for a call. You can put things together and be the one who invites others out. You can even call them up and see if they already have plans that you can tag along for.

Don't succumb to fears of coming across as needy or desperate. Remember that this is your commitment and you are willing to do whatever it takes to get out there and meet people. Remember that others may feel the same hesitation or apprehension that you feel when wanting to invite them out. What you put in is what you get back.

- **Don't get Offended if People don't seem Responsive:** Sometimes, others are preoccupied, busy, or thoughtless about attempting to hang out with you. This could lead to them never asking you to meet up and mean that you need to take the first step. Also, they may never think to invite you out if you don't take the initiative and get to know them better, first.

On a similar note, some individuals are really laid back and lax about getting back to you over text or e-mail. This doesn't mean that they are trying to ignore you or reject your attempts to get to know them. It can be a simple personality quality.

- **Don't get Hung up on Thinking it's Hard to Make Friends:** If you are not used to making attempts to meet friends, you might think of the whole experience as complicated and inconvenient. After all, a lot of times, all you have to do is meet someone you get along with and make an effort to see them multiple times. You also shouldn't think that you need to get to know them for a long time before thinking of them as a friend.

A quality you will notice in people who are very social is that they will use that word quite loosely with people. This doesn't mean that those connections are always deep or very personal bonds, but you can still enjoy their presence and gradually grow closer with time.

- **Remember that you Cannot be too Picky at First:** If you need friends and have been feeling very lonely, your very first priority should be starting from where you are. This means hanging out with anyone who gets along with you and appears to be interested in you as a person. This doesn't mean that the first few friends you make will be ideal in every way or end up as best friends, but there are a lot of benefits to just getting out there instead of staying at home alone.

  You can also remember that you will find it easier to meet new people when you already have a couple of friends. Plus, if you are just starting out with creating your first social circle, it can be hard to tell what you value in friends. The only way to find out is to meet as many as possible. A basic rule you can apply here is that if you seem to get along decently with a person, making the effort to get to know them more can let you know if they are a potential friend.

If you are more on the picky side with social relations, you can find plenty of reasons to hold yourself back from making friends. But once you force yourself to hang out with them anyway, you have already gotten past this block and might find that you enjoy their presence more than you expected. People can often surprise you in this way and this can lead to lifelong friendships.

- **Try not to be too Negative about the Process:** Plenty of research has shown that people who are solitary or lonely by nature have a tendency to have negative attitudes about other people, more so than people with a lot friends. People who are not as outgoing have the luxury of being more selective with who they want to spend time around.

If you find yourself wanting to look down on people you meet, you should make the effort to look past these urges.

- **Take Note of your Imagine of Yourself:** A negative self-image can also contribute to being judgmental about other people. Work on making sure that your image of yourself is realistic and healthy, and you will go a long way toward making good friends. If you don't have the highest opinion of yourself, you may find it difficult to be around people that are a lot like you since it can show you what you don't like about yourself.

  Try to take note of reasons why you might want to avoid new potential friends. It could turn out that you are giving up great opportunities to get to know nice people just because of your own insecurities.

- **Remember to Stay Persistent in the Process:** You may find that at times you join a hobby group or get introduced to a group of people with high hopes, and nothing seems to come of it. This may tempt you to become disheartened by the whole process and want to give up. It may lead you to think that you just don't get along with others or that they are rejecting you.

Do yourself, and others, a favor by giving the people more than one try. It's normal that the first time or two, you don't connect very well with people, but it can happen eventually if you make more efforts to hang out. If you find that a person declines your invite because they are busy that evening, don't allow this to make you give up on the whole process. Try it again later. You should never jump to assumptions about their attitudes toward you based on something like this.

With this process, it pays to only make positive assumptions. Even taking the initiative to invite someone out shows them that you like them and want to get to know them better. Just because they can't hang out that first time, but the invitation will put you into their mind for future events.

- **Stay Realistic about Expectations:** Remember that when you are just getting to know new people, you should stay realistic about how important you are to them. After all, they don't know you that well yet, and it's going to take some time to get closer with them. Remember that they probably already have friends and could be busier than you or occupied with other things. Don't expect that they will want to jump into hanging out every day with you right after you meet them for the first time. It could take a while to get closer to them.

At times, it won't end up being fruitful to try to get to know someone. It may appear promising at first, but then things could fizzle out after you meet up with them another couple of times. Either that, or they could be available the first time or two and then end up falling off the map soon after. This could be because they are busy with work, have a lot of friends already, or plenty of other reasons. You shouldn't take this personally and let it get you down. This is a common situation that everyone experiences.

If People Seem Uninterested in Getting to Know you More:

The idea of being the first to take initiative and not giving up right away can be all some people need to meet the perfect friends. Sometimes, even after taking initiative and persisting with people, you find that people still don't respond. There are a few things to keep in mind when this happens:

- **Stay as Patient as you can:** In an ideal world, you would find a great circle of friends very fast, even after moving somewhere completely new. You would meet your best buddy the first day after arriving to the new city or starting a new job. Unfortunately, life rarely works out this way. You will usually find that friendships take longer than that to form, but you should always stay with the process instead of giving up.

You may find that it takes a long time before you meet the right people who will be your close, lasting friends. Even after this, you may find that some months need to pass before you get to know them a lot better or see them often. Even after that, it could take years to develop into very close friends who you will have for life. Remember that it usually takes some time to shift from not having plans, to making consistent plans with one person all the time, to having them in your life permanently or constantly.

Chapter 5: Strengthening Existing Relationships

Friends are valuable to us in life, and we all need them. In a lot of situations, they are what saves us during the hard times and give us the strength to persevere. Whether you are going through a divorce, the loss of a loved one, or another huge shift in life, friends will come to your rescue and revive your hope in life. They will be there to give you advice, new perspectives, and more. They will provide you with courage and strength when you have none.

Part of, not only making friends, but strengthening existing bonds with friends, is knowing how to analyze people and carry yourself. A friendship is not something that is simply created and then lasts forever without effort. A friendship must be constantly rebuilt and worked on, which is what makes it so valuable to us. So, the question is, when undertaking the quest of understanding ourselves and others better, and attempting to strengthen our existing friendships, how can we deepen these bonds?

Here are some Surefire Ways to Strengthen the Important Bonds in your Life:

- **Make Sure you Stay Aware of your Friendships:** At times, we become so busy and preoccupied with family and life that we almost forget that our friendships exist. This means that we need to stay conscious of these people and remember that they won't exist forever. Maybe they are just a classmate or neighbor at one point, but that doesn't mean they won't become closer to us later. Remember that whoever you spend the most time with is who you are working on building real friendships with.

- **Never Take them for Granted:** Remember that being friends with someone is a choice you constantly make, not something you are obligated to do. This is what makes it so valuable and meaningful. If you do not stay aware of this fact and value the people who are close to you, they won't stay close for long, unfortunately.

In our busy modern society, everyone is moving constantly. If we don't make it a point to pay attention to our close friends, they will get further and further away from us until we are left wondering what ever happened to the people we held so dear at one point.

- **Look for Ways to Help your Friends in Times of Need:** Having friends is great because we can rely on them to be there, but this means we need to return the favor and always look for ways to help them out of hard times. The best time to be the best friend you can be is when your friend is going through a hard time.

This doesn't mean you need to take it upon yourself to solve all of their issues, because this can weigh on you in a negative way, but you can be a listening ear and a shoulder to cry on, if they need it. You can be there to help them with errands or meals, if they need it, as well.

At times, people who are going through hard or trying times are afraid to impose upon you, so they don't reach out. This is the perfect opportunity to be the first to extend the warm hand of friendship and find out how you can help them, without waiting for them to ask you for help.

- **Look for Ways to Improve your Friend's Lives:** You shouldn't only extend a warm hand of friendship to your close loved ones when they are going through something difficult. Search for ways to make their lives happier and more meaningful. Maybe they are busy with work but need to get something else done. This is the perfect chance to step in and do them a favor.

  Maybe they need a babysitter but haven't had a chance to call one. This is the perfect chance to do them a favor, without being asked. Always be looking for ways to help them out and make them even happier to be friends with you.

- **Never Forget Quality Time with your Friends:** Sure, this may seem obvious, but it's important to keep in mind. Family demands or work issues can take up a lot of our time. Daily schedules may seem like endless demanding to-do lists, but we must always make time to meet with our friends. We should set aside at least one day a week to spend time with them to keep the friendship growing and flourishing. Otherwise, we may lose them.

- **Make Sure to Stay in Touch all the Time:** Along with setting aside quality time to spend with your friends, you should make it a point to talk to them and catch up with them apart from this, as well. Not communicating with your friends enough will play a negative role on the relationship and must be kept in mind. We have the advantage in modern day of having devices which make it easy and simple to reach out to someone with a quick email or text. Stay in touch with your friends, even if it's a small message or quick phone call. This can make all the difference when it comes to your relationship.

- **Always be Supportive of their Aspirations:** You may find that your friends get lost sometimes, seem confused, or need advice. You must set aside time in your day to offer them the help they need. This is what friends are for. A lot of people in our lives are quick to laugh off someone's idea or passion, and friends should never be the ones who do this.

Friends should be there to listen to our ideas and give us encouragement when we need it. We should also be able to share our dreams with them and receive support back. If you want to make your friendships stronger and more lasting, you need to give them constructive, helpful advice that will be of value to their specific life path. There may be times that you find your friend's idea silly, but even then, you should help them make a list of pros and cons and find the best way to navigate their dream.

- **Remember how Important Friendship is:** The reason why we keep certain people around us month after month or year after year is because they matter to us in a significant way. Not having time is a terrible excuse to abandon your friendships. When something truly matters to you, you make the time, no matter what.

At times, we get overwhelmed and busy, but if your close relationships mean a lot to you, take the time to make them a top priority in your life. As soon as you do this, you will give yourself the permission to place friendship in front of other obligations that are, in reality, less important to you on a fundamental level. While issues or busy work schedules come and go, friendships can last forever.

At the end of life, it is not the hours we didn't work that we will look back upon with regret, but the time we didn't spend with the ones we love the most. Always keep in mind how important these bonds are.

- **Be Forgiving about their Faults:** It's natural that friends will get on your nerves at times with their habits or behavior. But, if they are a great friend, you should look past this for the sake of preserving the relationship. Everyone has their good and bad qualities, and true friendship embraces and accepts them all.

Sure, it may be hard, but to preserve the friendship, it's worth it to look past these qualities that annoy you.

- **Keep Expectations in Check:** You may find that when you observe your annoyance at a close friend, your anger is due to them defying an expectation you had of them that may have been unrealistic. We want our friends to call us every birthday, thank us for everything we do for them, and remember every important event in our lives, but fulfilling all of this is not always possible.

This kind of attitude can ruin a great friendship. Don't expect your friends to be perfect all the time. It's hard to find valuable friends, so once you do, keep your expectations in check and treat them fairly. It's worth it to save something that is so beneficial and worthwhile. If you treat them this way, they will return the favor.

Chapter 6: The dark side of human psychology – detecting liars, cheaters, and others alike

If only detecting liars was as easy as seeing if Pinocchio grow his nose, liars wouldn't exist in today's world.   Sadly this is not the case and they are found much often than you would think. Detecting hidden negative aspects of a person's character can be tough, but using human psychology and picking up certain verbal and non-verbal cues can influence your relationship with that person of interest.

Verbal and Nonverbal Cues

There are many different ways someone can detect a liar or a cheater. In fact, many of the cues that a person will give off if they are cheating on their partner or lying to someone are actually nonverbal. This is mostly because the majority of the way people communicate are through facial expression, body language, eye contact (or lack thereof) and tone of voice. Research shows that 97% of our commination is nonverbal, while only 7% is verbal. Remember the old saying "It's not so much what you say, but how you say it"? Well, that stands true in many different cases. You don't have to be a detective or private investigator to spot if someone is being untruthful or deceitful, you just need to learn how to pick up on a few things.

It is easiest to do this when you know the person intimately, yet it can also be the hardest simply because of the emotions that are tied into it. You can't be betrayed by an enemy. Yet, it is usually best to know the truth. One of the easiest ways to know if someone is cheating on you is by their behavior. There are times when, on the surface, the person you suspect is lying and/or cheating on you will act as if they are more in love with you. Many times, because people do not know the signs to look for, people get away with cheating and lying, at least for a while, because their spouse or significant other does not suspect there is a problem. On the contrary, the one who is being lied to might think that their relationship has never been better. The one who is being deceitful may perform outward acts of affection, such as buying presents or taking their partner places, as a way to deal with their immense feelings guilt. They do this in an attempt to justify their actions to themselves. They will usually then have thoughts like "I'm not that bad, look at all this awesome stuff I've been buying her lately! She's lucky to have someone like me around, no one else would do all this stuff for her."

This behavior will go on usually only until the other person feels there may be something going on and begins to ask questions. At this point, the one who is lying or cheating would become avoidant or hostile. In some cases, the person who is cheating and lying will go through both phases, first becoming avoidant in hopes that they can steer clear of conflict. If the questioning persists, they may then become hostile in an attempt to place the blame on the innocent partner, so that they do not need to accept the blame themselves.

During the avoidance phase, the lair or cheater will usually not be able to look you in the eye when you ask them a direct question related to their activity. There may be long pauses before an answer is given and answers are either very vague, or they may get nervous and give out too much information than is necessary for that particular question. Intimacy and physical touch usually suffers and may become nonexistent. They may have trouble sleeping and eating, and may become very irritable when you try to talk to them.

Another way to tell if someone is lying is if they are looking at you, and then in response to your question or statement, they look down and to the left. Later on, during the hostile phase, the person's tone of voice will most likely be harsh and accusing. People naturally become defensive if they are doing something wrong and someone, in turn, accuses them of that wrong action.

Conclusion

Thank you again for downloading this book!

I hope this book was able to help you to feel more confident in reading people, interacting with them, and expressing yourself to strangers and friends alike. People struggle with this aspect of life only because they don't have access to the right information. Now that you have read this guide, you're well on your way to becoming a master communicator with fewer and fewer misunderstandings and mistakes in interactions.

The next step is to test out the information you read in this book for yourself and see how well it works for you. If you follow the facts given in this guide, you should see an improvement in your ability to read others and communicate with them within a short period of time. You can then pass along this knowledge to others.

Don't forget that the way people seem to express themselves is not always telling of how they truly feel, and that culture plays a huge role in body language and what it means.

Finally, if you enjoyed this book, then I'd like to ask you for a favor, would you be kind enough to leave a review for this book on Amazon? It'd be greatly appreciated!

Thank you and good luck!